Slow Cooker Dishes

An Unmissable Recipe Collection For your Lunch

Donna Conway

implied. readers acknowledge that the author is not engaging in the rendering of legal, financial, medical or professional advice. the content within this book has been derived from various sources. please consult a licensed professional before attempting any techniques outlined in this book.

by reading this document, the reader agrees that under no circumstances is the author responsible for any losses, direct or indirect, which are incurred as a result of the use of information contained within this document, including, but not limited to, — errors, omissions, or inaccuracies.

Table of Contents

Cider-Braised Chicken

Preparation time: 10 minutes

Cooking time: 5 hours

Servings: 2 people

Ingredients:

- 4 chicken drumsticks
- 2 tablespoon of olive oil
- ½ cup of apple cider vinegar
- 1 tablespoon of balsamic vinegar
- 1 chili pepper, diced
- 1 yellow onion, minced
- Salt and black pepper- to taste

Directions:

1. Start by throwing all the ingredients into a bowl and mix them well. Marinate this chicken for 2 hours in the refrigerator.

2. Spread the chicken along with its marinade in the slow cooker. Cover it and cook for 5 hours on low. Serve warm.

Nutrition:

Calories: 311

Fat: 25.5g

Carbs: 1.4g

Protein: 18.4g

Chunky Chicken Salsa

Preparation time: 10 minutes

Cooking time: 6 hours

Servings: 2 people

Ingredients:

- 1 lb. chicken breast, skinless and boneless
- 1 cup of chunky salsa
- 3/4 teaspoon of cumin
- A pinch oregano
- Salt and black pepper- to taste

Directions:

1. Put all the fixings into the slow cooker and mix them well. Cover it and cook for 6 hours on low. Serve warm.

Nutrition: Calories: 541 Fat: 34g Carbs: 3.4g Protein: 20.3g

Dijon Chicken

Preparation time: 10 minutes

Cooking time: 6 hours

Servings: 4 people

Ingredients:

- 2 lbs. chicken thighs, skinless and boneless
- 3/4 cup of chicken stock
- 1/4 cup of lemon juice
- 2 tablespoon of extra virgin olive oil
- 3 tablespoon of Dijon mustard
- 2 tablespoons of Italian seasoning
- Salt and black pepper- to taste

Directions:

1. Put all the fixings into the slow cooker and mix them well. Cover it and cook for 6 hours on low. Serve warm.

Nutrition:

Calories: 398

Fat: 13.8g

Carbs: 3.6g

Protein: 51.8g

Chicken Dipped in Tomatillo Sauce

Preparation time: 10 minutes

Cooking time: 6 hours

Servings: 4 people

Ingredients:

- 1 lb. chicken thighs, skinless and boneless
- 2 tablespoon of extra virgin olive oil
- 1 yellow onion, sliced
- 1 garlic clove, crushed
- 4 oz. canned green chilies, diced
- 1 handful cilantro, diced
- 15 oz. cauliflower rice, already cooked
- 5 oz. tomatoes, diced
- 15 oz. cheddar cheese, grated
- 4 oz. black olives, pitted and diced
- Salt and black pepper- to taste

- 15 oz. canned tomatillos, diced

Directions:

1. Put all the fixings into the slow cooker and mix them well. Cover it and cook for 5 6 hours on low. Shred the slow-cooked chicken and return to the slow cooker. Mix well and garnish as desired. Serve warm.

Nutrition:

Calories: 427

Fat: 31.1g

Carbs: 9g

Protein: 23.5g

Mediterranean Beef Brisket

Preparation time: 20 minutes

Cooking time: 5 hours

Servings: 4 people

Ingredients:

- 3 lb. beef brisket, fat trimmed

- 3 teaspoons dried Italian seasoning

- 2 fennel bulbs, cored and sliced into wedges

- 14 oz. canned diced tomatoes with herbs

- 1 cup reduced-sodium beef stock

- ½ cup olives pitted

- 1 teaspoon lemon zest

- Salt and pepper to taste

- ¼ cup cold water mixed with 2 tablespoons all-purpose flour

Directions:

1. Sprinkle all sides of the beef brisket with 2 teaspoons Italian seasoning. Add to your slow cooker. Put the fennel on top of the beef.

2. In a bowl, mix the remaining Italian seasoning with the rest of the ingredients except the flour mixture. Pour over the beef and fennel. Cover the pot—cook on high for 5 hours.

3. Take the beef out of the pot and slice. Put it with the vegetables on a serving platter. Transfer the cooking liquid to a pan but discard the fat.

4. Stir in the flour mixture. Cook until the sauce has thickened. Pour the sauce over the beef and vegetables. Serve.

Nutrition: Calories: 254 Fat: 8g Carbs: 10g Protein: 35g

Spanish Beef

Preparation time: 10 minutes

Cooking time: 4 hours and 10 minutes

Servings: 4 people

Ingredients:

- 1 tablespoon olive oil

- 1 lb. beef stew meat

- salt and pepper to taste

- ½ cup onion, chopped

- 2 cloves garlic, crushed and minced

- 12 oz. sofrito

- ½ cup green olives, sliced in half

- 14 oz. canned diced tomatoes

- 2 cups potatoes, chopped

Directions:

1. Pour the oil into your pan over medium heat. Brown the beef in the pan. Season the beef with salt and pepper. Put the beef in your slow cooker.

2. Cook the onion and garlic in the beef drippings in the pan. Transfer to the slow cooker after 5 minutes. Stir in the rest of the ingredients. Cover the pot and set it to low—Cook for 4 hours.

Nutrition:

Calories: 560

Fat: 11.6g

Carbs: 13.6g

Protein: 19.6g

Beef with Artichokes & Olives

Preparation time: 10 minutes

Cooking time: 7 hours and 10 minutes

Servings: 4 people

Ingredients:

- 1 tablespoon olive oil

- 2 lb. beef stew meat

- 1 onion, diced

- 4 cloves garlic, chopped

- ½ cup Kalamata olives, chopped

- 14 oz artichoke hearts, drained and sliced in half.

- 14 oz canned diced tomatoes

- 15 oz canned tomato sauce

- 32 oz beef broth

- 1 bay leaf

- 1 teaspoon dried parsley

- 1 teaspoon dried oregano

- ½ teaspoon ground cumin

- 1 teaspoon dried basil

Directions:

1. Put the oil into a pan on medium heat. Cook the beef for 3 to 5 minutes per side. Transfer to your slow cooker. Stir in the rest of the ingredients. Cook on low for 7 hours. Discard the bay leaf before serving.

Nutrition:

Calories: 416

Fat: 26.2g

Carbs: 14.1g

Protein: 29.9g

Meatballs & Green Beans

Preparation time: 20 minutes

Cooking time: 8 hours

Servings: 4 people

Ingredients:

Green Beans:

- 1 lb. frozen green beans

- 1 onion, diced

- 2 cloves garlic, crushed and minced

- 15 oz. canned tomato sauce

- 30 oz. canned diced tomatoes

- ¼ teaspoon cayenne pepper

- 1 teaspoon cinnamon

- 1 teaspoon cumin

- Salt and pepper to taste

Meatballs:

- 1 lb. lean ground beef

- 1 tablespoon olive oil

- Salt and pepper to taste

- ¼ teaspoon cayenne pepper

- ½ teaspoon cinnamon

- ½ teaspoon allspice

- ½ teaspoon cumin

- ¼ cup plain breadcrumbs

- ¼ cup parsley, minced

Directions:

1. Mix all the green beans ingredients in your slow cooker. Mix all the fixings for the meatballs in a bowl.

2. Form meatballs from the ground beef mixture. Add the meatballs to the slow cooker. Coat with the sauce. Cook on low for 8 hours.

Nutrition: Calories: 103 Fat: 3.2g Carbs: 8.3g Protein: 11g

Beef in Balsamic Vinegar

Preparation time: 25 minutes

Cooking time: 8 hours

Servings: 4 people

Ingredients:

- 1 tablespoon olive oil

- 8 oz. mushrooms, sliced

- 1 onion, diced

- 2 lb. beef chuck steak, cut into cubes

- 1 cup beef stock

- 1 cup black olives, sliced

- 1 tablespoon capers

- ½ cup tomato sauce

- 14 oz. diced tomatoes

- ¼ cup balsamic vinegar

- 2 tablespoons fresh parsley, chopped

- 2 tablespoons fresh rosemary, chopped

- Salt and pepper to taste

Directions:

1. Pour the oil into your pan over medium heat. Cook the mushrooms for 5 minutes. Add the onions and cook for 5 more minutes. Transfer to the cooker.

2. Brown the beef in the pan for 12 to 15 minutes, turning once or twice. Put the beef in the slow cooker.

3. Pour the beef stock into the pan to deglaze. Scrape the brown bits and add them to the slow cooker. Stir in the rest of the ingredients. Cook on low for 8 hours.

Nutrition:

Calories: 368

Fat: 14.7g

Carbs: 9g

Protein: 48.9g

Mediterranean Pork Tenderloin

Preparation time: 10 minutes

Cooking time: 2 hours

Servings: 4 people

Ingredients:

- 4 cloves garlic, crushed and minced

- 1 cup chicken broth

- 1 tablespoon garam masala

- Salt and pepper to taste

- 16 oz. pork tenderloin, trimmed

- 1 cup couscous

- ½ cup raisins

- ½ cup almonds, sliced and toasted

- 2 tablespoons red wine vinegar

- ½ cup fresh parsley, minced

- ½ cup olive oil

Directions:

1. Add the garlic and broth to the slow cooker. In a bowl, mix the garam masala, salt, and pepper. Rub this mixture on both sides of the pork.

2. Add the pork to the slow cooker. Cook on low for 2 hours. Transfer the pork to a cutting board, then let rest for 2 minutes before slicing. Remove the fat off the cooking liquid in the pot.

3. Add the raisins and couscous and cook on high for 15 minutes. Add the almonds and mix well. In another bowl, combine the vinegar, oil, and parsley. Serve the pork with the couscous and vinaigrette.

Nutrition:

Calories: 682

Fat: 35.9g

Carbs: 52.2g

Protein: 39.9g

Mediterranean Pork Roast

Preparation time: 15 minutes

Cooking time: 6 hours

Servings: 4 people

Ingredients:

- 4 teaspoons Greek seasoning, divided

- 1 pork loin roast (boneless), fat trimmed

- 2 fennel bulbs, sliced

- 4 tomatoes, chopped

- ½ cup reduced-sodium chicken broth

- 2 tablespoons reduced-sodium chicken broth

- Salt and pepper to taste

- 2 teaspoons cornstarch

- 1 ½ teaspoon Worcestershire sauce

- ¼ cup black olives, chopped

Directions:

1. Sprinkle 1 teaspoon Greek seasoning on both sides of the pork. Add the fennel to the slow cooker. Put the pork on top.

2. Add the tomatoes around the pork. Pour ½ cup chicken broth into the slow cooker, then stir in the salt, pepper, and remaining Greek seasoning.

3. Set it to low and cook for 6 hours. Stir the remaining broth with the cornstarch and Worcestershire sauce. Put the sauce over the pork, then sprinkle with olives on top before serving.

Nutrition:

Calories: 213

Fat: 8.6g

Carbs: 8.5g

Protein: 24.9g

Pork Chops & Couscous

Preparation time: 10 minutes

Cooking time: 8 hours

Servings: 4 people

Ingredients:

- ¾ cup low-sodium chicken broth

- 2 tablespoons olive oil

- 2 ¼ teaspoons dried sage

- 1 teaspoon oregano

- 1 teaspoon basil

- ½ tablespoon garlic powder

- ½ tablespoon paprika

- ¼ teaspoon dried thyme

- ¼ teaspoon dried marjoram

- ¼ teaspoon dried rosemary

- 2 lb. pork chops, fat trimmed (boneless)

- 2 cups couscous, cooked

Directions:

1. Combine the chicken broth, olive oil, and spices in a bowl. Make slits on the pork chops. Pour the spice mixture into your slow cooker.

2. Put the pork and turn to coat evenly. Cook on low for 8 hours. Serve pork chops with couscous.

Nutrition:

Calories: 561

Fat: 32.1g

Carbs: 34.5g

Protein: 31.4g

Creamy Pork Chops with Potatoes

Preparation time: 10 minutes

Cooking time: 4 hours

Servings: 4 people

Ingredients:

- cooking spray
- 4 pork chops
- 6 potatoes, cubed
- 1 cup milk
- 1 packet dry ranch dressing mix
- garlic salt and pepper to taste
- 3 cups cream of onion soup

Directions:

1. Coat a slow cooker with oil. Arrange the potatoes inside the pot. Top with the pork chops. Mix the rest of the fixings in a bowl.

2. Pour this mixture over the pork chops and potatoes. Set it to high and cook for 4 hours. Pour the sauce over the pork chops and potatoes before serving.

Nutrition:

Calories: 488

Fat: 11g

Carbs: 57g

Protein: 36g

Mediterranean Pork Chops

Preparation time: 15 minutes

Cooking time: 6 hours

Servings: 4 people

Ingredients:

- 6 pork chops

- garlic salt and pepper to taste

- 2 teaspoons dried basil

- 1 teaspoon oregano

- 2 teaspoons paprika

- 3 tablespoons olive oil

- 4 tablespoons balsamic vinegar

- 8 oz. chicken broth

- 1 cup carrot, cubed

- 1 cups potato, cubed

Directions:

1. Coat the slow cooker with cooking spray. Sprinkle both sides of the pork chops with garlic salt, pepper, basil, oregano, and paprika.

2. Transfer to the slow cooker. Mix the balsamic vinegar and olive oil. Pour into the pot. Pour in the chicken broth. Stir in the carrots and potatoes. Cook on low for 6 hours. Serve.

Nutrition:

Calories: 344

Fat: 27.2g

Carbs: 4.8g

Protein: 19.3g

Greek Shredded Beef

Preparation time: 15 minutes

Cooking time: 4 hours

Servings: 4 people

Ingredients:

- 2 lb. beef chuck roast, fat trimmed and cubed
- Salt to taste
- 1 cup onion, chopped
- ¾ cup red bell pepper, chopped
- ¾ cup carrots, chopped
- 14 oz. canned roasted tomatoes
- 2 tablespoons red wine vinegar
- 1 tablespoon garlic, crushed and minced
- 1 tablespoon Italian seasoning blend
- ½ tablespoon dried red pepper

Directions:

1. Season the beef chuck roast with salt. Put the beef cubes in the slow cooker. Sprinkle the onion, bell pepper, and carrots on top.

2. In a bowl, mix the rest of the ingredients and pour into the pot—cook on high for 4 hours. Shred with the beef. Serve with salad or whole wheat bread.

Nutrition:

Calories: 589

Fat: 42.1g

Carbs: 8.6g

Protein: 40.8g

Pork with Sweet Potatoes & Mushrooms

Preparation time: 15 minutes

Cooking time: 5 hours

Servings: 2 people

Ingredients:

- 1 lb. pork tenderloin, diced

- 1 yellow bell pepper, sliced

- 1 zucchini, sliced into rounds

- 1 sweet potato, cubed

- 1 tablespoon olive oil

- 2 onions, sliced

- 1 clove garlic, minced

- ¼ cup tomato sauce

- 2 cups pork broth

- 1 teaspoon dried oregano

- Pepper to taste

- 1 cup mushrooms

Directions:

1. Put the pork, bell pepper, zucchini, and sweet potato into the slow cooker. Put the oil and cook the onion for 2 minutes in a pan over medium heat.

2. Stir in the garlic and cook for 2 minutes. Transfer the onion and garlic to the slow cooker. In the same pan, pour in the tomato sauce and broth.

3. Season with pepper and oregano. Boil and then move to the slow cooker. Mix everything. Cook on low for 3 hours. Stir in the mushrooms and cook on low for another 1 hour.

Nutrition:

Calories: 572

Fat: 17.1g

Carbs: 34.6g

Protein: 70g

Moroccan Lamb

Preparation time: 15 minutes

Cooking time: 4 hours and 15 minutes

Servings: 4 people

Ingredients:

- 1 onion, chopped

- 3 cloves garlic, chopped

- 6 potatoes, cubed

- 3 carrots, sliced into cubes

- 2 lb. lamb leg, cut into cubes

- ½ cup dried apricots

- 1 bay leaf

- 1 cinnamon stick

- ½ teaspoon ground ginger

- 1 teaspoon Moroccan spice blend

- 1 ½ teaspoon ground allspice

- 6 tomatoes from the can slice in half

- 3 cups reduced-sodium beef stock

- 15 oz. canned chickpeas

Directions:

1. Put the olive oil and cook the onion, garlic, potatoes, and carrots for 5 minutes in a pan over medium heat. Season with salt and pepper.

2. Transfer the vegetables to the slow cooker. Add the lamb and brown on both sides, then put the apricots, bay leaf, cinnamon stick, and spices.

3. Stir in the tomatoes. Bring to a boil for 5 minutes. Move it to the slow cooker—cook on high for 4 hours. Serve.

Nutrition:

Calories: 502

Fat: 9.7g

Carbs: 65.4g

Protein: 43.5g

Mediterranean Lamb Chops

Preparation time: 10 minutes

Cooking time: 8 hours

Servings: 4 people

Ingredients:

- 4 lamb shoulder chops, fat trimmed

- 2 onions, sliced

- 4 cloves garlic, sliced

- 1 tablespoon paprika

- 2 cups canned tomatoes

- 1 tablespoon tomato paste

- 2 sprigs rosemary

- 1 pack frozen mixed vegetables

Directions:

1. Combine all the ingredients except vegetables in the slow cooker. Cook on low for 7 hours. Stir in the vegetables. Cook for another 1 hour. Pour the sauce over the lamb chops before serving.

Nutrition:

Calories: 307

Fat: 8.9g

Carbs: 20.4g

Protein: 35.8g

Greek Leg of Lamb

Preparation time: 20 minutes

Cooking time: 4 hours and 6 minutes

Servings: 4 people

Ingredients:

- 3 lb. leg of lamb

- Salt and pepper to taste

- 4 tablespoons olive oil, divided

- 12 cloves garlic

- 1 tablespoon freshly squeezed lemon juice

- ¾ teaspoons sweet paprika

- 2 teaspoons fresh thyme, chopped

- 1 teaspoon dried oregano

- 2 teaspoons dried rosemary

- 1 lb. onion, peeled

- ½ cup reduced-sodium beef broth

- 1 cup dry red wine

- Chopped parsley

Directions:

1. Flavor both sides of the lamb with salt plus pepper to taste. Pour half of the olive oil into a pan over medium heat.

2. Add the lamb and cook for 3 minutes per side. After cooking, make several slits on the lamb. Insert garlic clove in each slit.

3. In a bowl, mix the lemon juice, paprika, thyme, oregano, and rosemary. Rub mixture all over the lamb. Add the lamb to the slow cooker.

4. Top with the onion and pour in the broth and wine. Seal the pot and cook on high for 4 hours.

Nutrition: Calories179 Fat: 12.9g Carbs: 13.2g Protein: 5.1g

Beef Tenderloin with Rosemary

Preparation time: 15 minutes

Cooking time: 8 hours

Servings: 4 people

Ingredients:

- 1 tbsp of tallow

- 3 ½ lbs. beef tenderloin roast

- Salt and freshly ground pepper, to taste

- 3 cloves of garlic finely chopped

- 6 fresh rosemary sprigs chopped

- 1/4 cup of extra-virgin olive oil

- 1/4 cup of mustard

- 1 cup of white wine or water

Directions:

1. Coat your slow cooker with tallow. Season beef with salt and pepper, and place in a slow cooker.

2. Sprinkle the rosemary evenly over the meat. In a bowl, combine olive oil, mustard, wine, and salt and pepper. Pour the mixture over meat and toss to mix well.

3. Cook on high within 4 hours or low heat for 6 to 8 hours. Remove the beef on a working surface and allow it to cool for 10 minutes. Slice and serve.

Nutrition:

Calories: 477

Carbs: 3g

Fat: 39g

Protein: 28g

Braised Round Steak with Rosemary

Preparation time: 15 minutes

Cooking time: 8 hours

Servings: 4 people

Ingredients:

- 1 tbsp of beef tallow

- 2 lbs. of beef cheeks cut into slices

- 2 spring onions finely sliced

- 1/2 cup of fresh celery finely chopped

- 1 clove of garlic minced

- 2 bay leaves

- 1 tbsp of dried rosemary (or fresh)

- salt and ground black pepper to taste

- 2 to 3 cloves (whole)

- 1 cup of red wine

- 1 cup of water

Directions:

1. Add tallow in your slow cooker. Add the beef slices and all remaining ingredients (except red wine).

2. Pour red wine and water into a slow cooker and toss to combine well—cover and cook on high within 4 hours or low for 8 hours. Serve hot.

Nutrition:

Calories: 94

Carbs: 15g

Fat: 2g

Protein: 8g

Braised Beef Tenderloin with Broccoli and Sesame

Preparation time: 15 minutes

Cooking time: 4 hours & 30 minutes

Servings: 4 people

Ingredients:

- 2 lbs. of beef tenderloin sliced

- 1 cup of bone broth

- 1/4 cup of coconut aminos

- 2 tbsp of olive oil

- 1/4 cup of granulated stevia sweetener

- 3 cups of broccoli flowerets

- Salt and ground black pepper to taste

- 3 tbsp of sesame seeds

Directions:

1. Place the beef meat directly on the bottom of the slow cooker. Combine the coconut aminos, olive oil, and stevia sweetener.

2. Pour the mixture evenly over the beef. Cook on high within 3 to 4 hours. Open the lid and add broccoli florets—season with salt and pepper.

3. Cook on high for 30 minutes. Sprinkle with sesame seeds and serve hot.

Nutrition:

Calories: 360

Carbs: 27g

Fat: 15g

Protein: 28g

Old Ranch Pork Chops

Preparation time: 15 minutes

Cooking time: 4 hours & 10 minutes

Servings: 4 people

Ingredients:

- 2 lbs. of pork chops

- 3/4 cup of beer

- 3/4 tsp of cumin

- 1/2 tsp of caraway

- 2 tbsp of olive oil

- salt and ground black pepper to taste

- 1 tbsp of lard softened

Directions:

1. In a bowl, stir bear, cumin, caraway, salt, pepper, and olive oil. Put the pork chops in a large container and

pour the beer mixture; toss to combine well, and refrigerate for 3 hours.

2. Add softened lard to your slow cooker. Remove the chops from marinade and place in a slow cooker.

3. Pour a little marinade and cover. Cook on high heat for 4 hours. Baste with marinade occasionally. Serve hot.

Nutrition:

Calories: 248

Carbs: 5g

Fat: 12g

Protein: 27g

Lamb Shanks with Celery Root

Preparation time: 15 minutes

Cooking time: 9 hours

Servings: 4 people

Ingredients:

- 4 lamb shanks

- 16 oz sliced mushrooms

- 1 large carrot, diced

- 1 medium onion

- 1 large celery root

- 1 tbsp fresh chopped rosemary

- 2 tbsp extra virgin olive oil

- 1 cup dry red wine

- 3 tbsp Dijon mustard

- 1 tsp balsamic vinegar

- salt, black pepper

- 1 tbsp chopped parsley

- 4 large cloves garlic

Directions:

1. Place all ingredients in your slow cooker. Close and cook on low for 8 to 9 hours. Serve hot.

Nutrition:

Calories: 416

Carbs: 3g

Fat: 30g

Protein: 45g

Bacon Omelet

Preparation time: 15 minutes

Cooking time: 2 hours

Servings: 4 people

Ingredients:

- 1 tbsp of lard

- 1 lb. bacon finely sliced or chopped

- 1 green onion, finely chopped

- 1 bell pepper, diced

- 8 eggs from free-range chickens, beaten

- 1 pinch of crushed red paprika

- Salt and the ground black pepper to taste

Directions:

1. Grease the bottom of your slow cooker with lard. Add bacon, green onion, and bell pepper in a slow cooker.

2. In a bowl, whisk the eggs with the pinch of crushed paprika and salt and pepper to taste. Slowly pour the egg mixture over bacon and onions - do not stir.

3. Cover and cook on high within 2 hours. Remove the omelet from the slow cooker and allow it to rest for 5 minutes before slicing. Serve.

Nutrition:

Calories: 377

Carbs: 7g

Fat: 31g

Protein: 17g

Creamy Corn

Preparation time: 15 minutes

Cooking time: 2 hours

Servings: 4 people

Ingredients:

- 1 cup whole milk

- 16 oz. frozen corn kernels

- 2 tablespoons granulated sugar

- 1/4 cup all-purpose flour

- 2 large eggs beaten

- 1/2 teaspoon kosher salt

- 2 tablespoons unsalted butter

Directions:

1. In a 3 to 5-quart slow cooker, add all ingredients and mix to blend. Cover and cook for 1 to 2 hours on high or until the corn is smooth and thickened. Serve.

Nutrition:

Calories: 296

Carbs: 45g

Fat: 11g

Protein: 10g

Sweet Potatoes with Marshmallows

Preparation time: 15 minutes

Cooking time: 7 hours & 30 minutes

Servings: 4 people

Ingredients:

- 3/4 cup brown sugar
- 5 large sweet potatoes, cut into a 1-inch cube
- 1/4 cup butter melted
- 1 teaspoon ground nutmeg
- 1 teaspoon ground cinnamon
- 1/2 teaspoon kosher salt
- 3 cups miniature marshmallows
- 1/2 cup orange juice

Directions:

1. In a 4 to 6-quart slow cooker, put the sweet potatoes, brown sugar, butter, cinnamon, nutmeg, and salt on the bottom.

2. Cover and cook within 6 to 7 hours on low or 3 to 4 hours on high. Mash the sweet potatoes using your potato masher. Add orange juice to the mix.

3. Cover the top with marshmallows, cover with mashed sweet potatoes, and cook for an additional 20 to 30 minutes. Serve.

Nutrition:

Calories: 531

Fat: 6g

Carbs: 117g

Protein: 5g

Green Beans and Bacon

Preparation time: 15 minutes

Cooking time: 8 hours

Servings: 4 people

Ingredients:

- 29 oz. canned green beans

- 12 oz. center-cut bacon

- 1/2 cup real maple syrup

- 1 medium yellow onion chopped

- 1/4 cup brown sugar

Directions:

1. Just heat the bacon and onion in a saucepan until the bacon is cooked. Drain and empty the green beans into a 5-quart or larger slow cooker.

2. On top of the green beans, add the bacon, onion, and drippings. Put the brown sugar and maple syrup in the mixture and combine well—cover and cook within 6 to 8 hours on low or within 4 to 5 hours on high. Serve.

Nutrition:

Calories: 185

Fat: 9g

Carbs: 17g

Protein: 12g

Chunky Applesauce

Preparation time: 15 minutes

Cooking time: 6 hours

Servings: 4 people

Ingredients:

- 1 cup granulated sugar
- 3 pounds apples peeled, slice into large chunks
- 1 teaspoon ground cloves
- 2 teaspoons ground cinnamon
- 1 cup of water

Directions:

1. Put all the ingredients and mix to combine in a 6-quart or larger slow cooker. Cover and cook for 2 hours on high, then turn down to low and cook 4 to 6 hours or until tender. Mash the apples using a potato masher.

2. Stir in more sugar or honey, if necessary, while the applesauce is still warm. Add in tiny amounts until you achieve the perfect sweetness. Serve hot or refrigerate for up to 1 week.

Nutrition:

Calories: 139

Fat: 0.3g

Carbs: 36g

Protein: 0.3g

Parmesan Garlic Potatoes

Preparation time: 15 minutes

Cooking time: 5 hours

Servings: 4 people

Ingredients:

- 3 tablespoons unsalted butter melted
- 3 pounds baby potatoes washed and halved
- 1/2 teaspoon dried oregano
- 2 tablespoons olive oil
- 4 cloves garlic minced
- 1/2 teaspoon dried basil
- 1/4 teaspoon kosher salt
- 1/4 teaspoon freshly ground black pepper
- 1/2 teaspoon dried dill
- 1/2 cup parmesan cheese grated

Directions:

1. In a dish, toss the melted butter, olive oil, and minced garlic with the halved potatoes. Attach a 5-quart or larger slow cooker to the potatoes.

2. Mix dry seasoning (oregano, basil, dill, salt, and pepper) in another tub. Sprinkle the seasoning with the potatoes and toss gently.

3. Cook within 4 to 5 hours on low or 2 to 3 hours on high. Until serving, remove the potatoes from the slow cooker and sprinkle them with parmesan cheese.

Nutrition:

Calories: 191

Fat: 16g

Carbs: 3g

Protein: 8g

Coconut-Pecan Sweet Potatoes

Preparation time: 15 minutes

Cooking time: 5 hours

Servings: 4 people

Ingredients:

- 1/2 cup chopped pecans

- 4 pounds sweet potatoes, diced

- 1/2 cup butter melted

- 1/3 cup granulated sugar

- 1/2 cup unsweetened flaked coconut

- 1/3 cup brown sugar packed

- 1/4 teaspoon kosher salt

- 1/2 teaspoon pure vanilla extract

Directions:

1. Put the sweet potatoes in a slow cooker of 5 quarts or greater. Mix the pecans, coconut, melted butter sugar, vanilla extract, and salt in a dish.

2. Put the pecan mixture and toss it with the sweet potatoes in the slow cooker—cover and cook within 4 to 5 hours on low.

Nutrition:

Calories: 307

Fat: 16g

Carbs: 42g

Protein: 3g

Sugar Carrots with Ginger

Preparation time: 15 minutes

Cooking time: 6 hours

Servings: 4 people

Ingredients:

- 7 whole carrots sliced into 1/4-inch slices

- 1/4 cup brown sugar

- 3 tablespoons fresh ginger, minced

- 1/4 cup butter

- 1/4 cup orange juice

Directions:

1. Clean and remove the carrots and slice them into 1/4-inch pieces. Add carrots, ginger, orange juice, brown sugar, and butter to a 4-quart slow cooker.

2. Cover and cook for 1 hour. To ensure no clumps of brown sugar, remove the lid from the slow cooker and whisk in the carrot mixture.

3. Cover the slow cooker, adjust the temperature to low, and cook for an extra 4 to 5 hours or until the carrots hit the perfect tenderness amount. Serve.

Nutrition:

Calories: 221

Fat: 12g

Carbs: 29g

Protein: 1g

Sweet Acorn Squash

Preparation time: 15 minutes

Cooking time: 3 hours

Servings: 4 people

Ingredients:

- 2 tablespoons Butter
- 1 medium Acorn Squash, cut in half
- 2 tablespoons Brown Sugar

Directions:

1. By cutting each of them in half and scooping out the seeds and pulp, prepare your acorn squashes. Place a 4 quart or larger slow cooker with acorn squash halves skin-side down.

2. Score the inside of the squash all over the flesh with a sharp kitchen knife, being careful not to pierce the

skin. Divide the butter and brown sugar equally between the two halves of the squash.

3. Cover and cook on high within 3 hours or until the squash's flesh is soft and tender. Serve.

Nutrition:

Calories: 124

Fat: 6g

Protein: 1g

Carbs: 18g

Sweet Potatoes with Orange

Preparation time: 15 minutes

Cooking time: 6 hours

Servings: 4 people

Slow cooker size: 6-quart

Ingredients:

- 4 medium sweet potatoes

- 2 tablespoons orange zest

- 1/4 cup water or orange juice

- salt & pepper to taste

- 1/2 cup butter or dairy-free margarine

Directions:

1. Break the sweet potatoes lengthwise into quarters and then into large chunks. In a 6-quart slow cooker, add the sweet potatoes, water, and orange zest.

2. Cover and cook within 2 to 3 hours on high or 4 to 6 hours on low or until the sweet potatoes are easily fork-pierced.

3. Use a potato masher right in the slow cooker to mix up the sweet potatoes; add butter, salt, and pepper to taste. Serve.

Nutrition:

Calories: 237

Fat: 16g

Carbs: 23g

Protein: 2g

Veggie and Garbanzo Mix

Preparation time: 10 minutes

Cooking time: 6 hours

Servings: 4 people

Ingredients:

- 15 oz. canned garbanzo beans, drained
- 3 cups cauliflower florets
- 1 cup green beans
- 1 cup carrot, sliced
- 14 oz. veggie stock
- ½ cup onion, chopped
- 2 teaspoons curry powder
- ¼ cup basil, chopped
- 14 oz. of coconut milk

Directions:

1. In your slow cooker, mix beans with cauliflower, green beans, carrot, onion, stock, curry powder, basil,

and milk, stir, cover, and cook on low for 6 hours. Stir veggie mix again, divide between plates and serve as a side dish.

Nutrition:

Calories: 219

Fat: 5g

Carbs: 32g

Protein: 7g

Mushrooms and Sausage Mix

Preparation time: 10 minutes

Cooking time: 2 hours and 30 minutes

Servings: 4 people

Ingredients:

- ½ cup butter, melted

- 1-pound pork sausage, ground

- ½ pound mushrooms, sliced

- 6 celery ribs, chopped

- 2 yellow onions, chopped

- 2 garlic cloves, minced

- 1 tablespoon sage, chopped

- 1 cup cranberries, dried

- ½ cup cauliflower florets, chopped

- ½ cup veggie stock

Directions:

1. Heat-up a pan with the butter over medium-high heat, add sausage, stir, cook for a couple of minutes and transfer to your slow cooker.

2. Add mushrooms, celery, onion, garlic, sage, cranberries, cauliflower, stock, stir, cover, and cook on high for 2 hours and 30 minutes. Divide between plates and serve as a side dish.

Nutrition:

Calories: 200

Fat: 3g

Carbs: 9g

Protein: 4g

Glazed Baby Carrots

Preparation time: 10 minutes

Cooking time: 6 hours

Servings: 4 people

Ingredients:

- ½ cup peach preserves
- ½ cup butter, melted
- 2 pounds baby carrots
- 2 tablespoon sugar
- 1 teaspoon vanilla extract
- A pinch of salt and black pepper
- A bit of nutmeg, ground
- ½ teaspoon cinnamon powder
- 2 tablespoons water

Directions:

1. Put baby carrots in your slow cooker, add butter, peach preserves, sugar, vanilla, salt, pepper, nutmeg, cinnamon, and water, toss well, cover, and cook on low for 6 hours. Divide between plates and serve as a side dish.

Nutrition:

Calories: 283

Fat: 14g

Carbs: 28g

Protein: 3g

Buttery Mushrooms

Preparation time: 10 minutes

Cooking time: 4 hours

Servings: 4 people

Ingredients:

- 1 yellow onion, chopped
- 1 pound's mushrooms, halved
- ½ cup butter, melted
- 1 teaspoon Italian seasoning
- Salt and black pepper to the taste
- 1 teaspoon sweet paprika

Directions:

1. In your slow cooker, mix mushrooms with onion, butter, Italian seasoning, salt, pepper, and paprika,

toss, cover, and cook on low within 4 hours. Divide between plates and serve as a side dish.

Nutrition:

Calories: 120

Fat: 6g

Carbs: 8g

Protein: 4g

Cauliflower Rice and Spinach

Preparation time: 10 minutes

Cooking time: 3 hours

Servings: 4 people

Ingredients:

- 2 garlic cloves, minced

- 2 tablespoons butter, melted

- 1 yellow onion, chopped

- ¼ teaspoon thyme, dried

- 3 cups veggie stock

- 20 oz. spinach, chopped

- 6 oz. coconut cream

- Salt and black pepper to the taste

- 2 cups cauliflower rice

Directions:

1. Heat-up a pan with the butter over medium heat, add onion, stir and cook for 4 minutes. Add garlic, thyme, and stock, stir, cook for 1 minute more, and transfer to your slow cooker.

2. Add spinach, coconut cream, cauliflower rice, salt, and pepper, stir a bit, cover and cook on high for 3 hours. Divide between plates and serve as a side dish.

Nutrition:

Calories: 200

Fat: 4g

Carbs: 8g

Protein: 2g

Maple Sweet Potatoes

Preparation time: 10 minutes

Cooking time: 5 hours

Servings: 4 people

Ingredients:

- 4 sweet potatoes, halved and sliced

- 1 cup walnuts, chopped

- ½ cup cherries, dried and chopped

- ½ cup maple syrup

- ¼ cup apple juice

- A pinch of salt

Directions:

1. Arrange sweet potatoes in your slow cooker, add walnuts, dried cherries, maple syrup, apple juice, and a pinch of salt, toss a bit, cover, and cook on low for 5 hours. Divide between plates and serve as a side dish.

Nutrition: Calories: 271 Fat: 6g Carbs: 26g Protein: 6g

Sweet Potato Mash

Preparation time: 10 minutes

Cooking time: 5 hours

Servings: 4 people

Ingredients:

- 2 pounds sweet potatoes, peeled and sliced

- 1 tablespoon cinnamon powder

- 1 cup apple juice

- 1 teaspoon nutmeg, ground

- ¼ teaspoon cloves, ground

- ½ teaspoon allspice

- 1 tablespoon butter, melted

Directions:

1. In your slow cooker, mix sweet potatoes with cinnamon, apple juice, nutmeg, cloves, and allspice,

stir, cover, and cook on low within 5 hours. Mash using a potato masher, add butter, whisk well, divide between plates and serve as a side dish.

Nutrition:

Calories: 111

Fat: 2g

Carbs: 16g

Protein: 3g

Dill Cauliflower Mash

Preparation time: 10 minutes

Cooking time: 5 hours

Servings: 4 people

Ingredients:

- 1 cauliflower head, florets separated
- 1/3 cup dill, chopped
- 6 garlic cloves
- 2 tablespoons butter, melted
- A pinch of salt and black pepper

Directions:

1. Put cauliflower in your slow cooker, add dill, garlic, and water to cover cauliflower, cover, and cook on high for 5 hours.

2. Drain cauliflower and dill, add salt, pepper, and butter, mash using a potato masher, whisk well and serve as a side dish.

Nutrition:

Calories: 187

Fat: 4g

Carbs: 12g

Protein: 3g

Eggplant and Kale Mix

Preparation time: 10 minutes

Cooking time: 2 hours

Servings: 4 people

Ingredients:

- 14 oz. canned roasted tomatoes and garlic

- 4 cups eggplant, cubed

- 1 yellow bell pepper, chopped

- 1 red onion, cut into medium wedges

- 4 cups kale leaves

- 2 tablespoons olive oil

- 1 teaspoon mustard

- 3 tablespoons red vinegar

- 1 garlic clove, minced

- Salt and black pepper to the taste

- ½ cup basil, chopped

Directions:

1. In your slow cooker, mix the eggplant with tomatoes, bell pepper, and onion, toss, cover, and cook on high for 2 hours.

2. Add kale, toss, cover slow cooker and leave aside for now. In a bowl, mix oil with vinegar, mustard, garlic, salt, and pepper and whisk well. Add this over eggplant mix, add basil, toss, divide between plates and serve as a side dish.

Nutrition:

Calories: 251

Fat: 9g

Carbs: 34g

Protein: 8g

Thai Side Salad

Preparation time: 10 minutes

Cooking time: 3 hours

Servings: 4 people

Ingredients:

- 8 oz. yellow summer squash, peeled and roughly chopped
- 12 oz. zucchini, halved and sliced
- 2 cups button mushrooms, quartered
- 1 red sweet potato, chopped
- 2 leeks, sliced
- 2 tablespoons veggie stock
- 2 garlic cloves, minced
- 2 tablespoon Thai red curry paste
- 1 tablespoon ginger, grated
- 1/3 cup coconut milk
- ¼ cup basil, chopped

Directions:

1. In your slow cooker, mix zucchini with summer squash, mushrooms, red pepper, leeks, garlic, stock, curry paste, ginger, coconut milk, and basil, toss, cover, and cook on low for 3 hours. Stir your Thai mix one more time, divide between plates and serve as a side dish.

Nutrition:

Calories: 69

Fat: 2g

Carbs: 8g

Protein: 2g

Mint Farro Pilaf

Preparation time: 10 minutes

Cooking time: 4 hours

Servings: 2 people

Ingredients:

- ½ tablespoon balsamic vinegar
- ½ cup whole grain farro
- A pinch of salt and black pepper
- 1 cup chicken stock
- ½ tablespoon olive oil
- 1 tablespoon green onions, chopped
- 1 tablespoon mint, chopped

Directions:

1. In your slow cooker, mix the farro with the vinegar and the other ingredients, toss, cook on low within 4 hours. Divide between plates and serve.

Nutrition: Calories: 162 Fat: 3g Carbs: 9g Protein: 4g

Parmesan Rice

Preparation time: 10 minutes

Cooking time: 2 hours and 30 minutes

Servings: 2 people

Ingredients:

- 1 cup of rice

- 2 cups chicken stock

- 1 tablespoon olive oil

- 1 red onion, chopped

- 1 tablespoon lemon juice

- Salt and black pepper to the taste

- 1 tablespoon parmesan, grated

Directions:

1. In your slow cooker, mix the rice with the stock, oil, and the rest of the fixing, toss, cook on high for 2

hours and 30 minutes. Divide between plates and serve as a side dish.

Nutrition:

Calories: 162

Fat: 4g

Carbs: 29g

Protein: 6g

Lemon Artichokes

Preparation time: 10 minutes

Cooking time: 3 hours

Servings: 2 people

Ingredients:

- 1 cup veggie stock

- 2 medium artichokes, trimmed

- 1 tablespoon lemon juice

- 1 tablespoon lemon zest, grated

- Salt to the taste

Directions:

1. In your slow cooker, mix the artichokes with the stock and the rest of the fixing, toss, cook on low for 3 hours. Divide artichokes between plates and serve as a side dish.

Nutrition: Calories: 100 Fat: 2g Carbs: 10g Protein: 4g

Italian Eggplant

Preparation time: 10 minutes

Cooking time: 2 hours

Servings: 2 people

Ingredients:

- 2 small eggplants, roughly cubed
- ½ cup heavy cream
- Salt and black pepper to the taste
- 1 tablespoon olive oil
- A pinch of hot pepper flakes
- 2 tablespoons oregano, chopped

Directions:

1. In your slow cooker, mix the eggplants, cream, and the rest of the fixing, toss, and cook on high within 2 hours. Divide between plates and serve as a side dish.

Nutrition: Calories: 132 Fat: 4g Carbs: 12g Protein: 3g

Cabbage and Onion Mix

Preparation time: 10 minutes

Cooking time: 2 hours

Servings: 2 people

Ingredients:

- 1 and ½ cups green cabbage, shredded

- 1 cup red cabbage, shredded

- 1 tablespoon olive oil

- 1 red onion, sliced

- 2 spring onions, chopped

- ½ cup tomato paste

- ¼ cup veggie stock

- 2 tomatoes, chopped

- 2 jalapenos, chopped

- 1 tablespoon chili powder

- 1 tablespoon chives, chopped

- A pinch of salt and black pepper

Directions:

1. Grease your slow cooker with the oil and mix the cabbage with the onion, spring onions, and the other ingredients inside. Toss, and cook on high within 2 hours. Divide between plates and serve as a side dish.

Nutrition:

Calories: 211

Fat: 3g

Carbs: 6g

Protein: 8g

Balsamic Okra Mix

Preparation time: 10 minutes

Cooking time: 2 hours

Servings: 4 people

Ingredients:

- 2 cups okra, sliced

- 1 cup cherry tomatoes, halved

- 1 tablespoon olive oil

- ½ teaspoon turmeric powder

- ½ cup canned tomatoes, crushed

- 2 tablespoons balsamic vinegar

- 2 tablespoons basil, chopped

- 1 tablespoon thyme, chopped

Directions:

1. In your slow cooker, mix the okra with the tomatoes, crushed tomatoes, and the rest of the fixing, toss, put the lid on and cook on high for 2 hours. Divide between plates and serve as a side dish.

Nutrition:

Calories: 233

Fat: 12g

Carbs: 8g

Protein: 4g

Chicken Curry

Preparation time: 15 minutes

Cooking time: 6 hours

Servings: 4 people

Ingredients:

- 2 pounds of chicken breasts/thighs
- 2 cups full fat coconut milk
- 6 cups, your choice, fresh vegetables
- 1 tablespoon cumin
- 1 cup tomato sauce
- 2 teaspoons ground ginger
- 2 teaspoons ground coriander
- 1 teaspoon cinnamon
- 2 teaspoons garlic powder
- 1 cup of water
- ½ teaspoon cayenne pepper
- pinch of salt and fresh ground pepper, each

Directions:

1. Rinse the chicken, pat dry. Dice the vegetables and chicken into chunks. Place all the fixings in your slow cooker.

2. Add the coconut milk, tomatoes, and spices. Add the cup of water. Cover and cook on low within 6 hours. Serve hot—side with rice or greens.

Nutrition:

Calories: 515

Fat: 29.3g

Carb 23.2g

Protein: 39.8g

Stuffed Chicken Breasts

Preparation time: 15 minutes

Cooking time: 6 hours

Servings: 2-4 people

Ingredients:

- 6 boneless chicken breasts

- 1/3 cup feta cheese, crumbled

- 1-2 teaspoons fresh oregano

- pinch of salt, fresh ground pepper, each

- 1 tablespoon olive oil

- ½ onion, diced

- 2 teaspoons minced garlic

- ¾ cup fresh spinach

- juice of 1 lemon

- 2 pepperoncini peppers

- ½ red pepper, diced

- 1 cup chicken stock

- ½ cup white wine

Directions:

1. Rinse the chicken, pat dry. Slice the chicken breasts ¾ open. Leave them attached. In a large bowl, combine feta cheese, oregano, salt, and pepper.

2. In a large skillet, heat the olive oil. Add the onion, cook 2 minutes, then put the garlic, cook 1 minute. Add the spinach. Heat until the spinach wilts.

3. Add the spinach batter to the bowl with feta cheese. Add the lemon juice, pepperoncini peppers, red pepper. Stir to combine.

4. Stuff the chicken breasts with the mixture. Place them in the slow cooker. Pour in chicken stock and wine—cover and cook on for 6 hours, then serve hot—side with salad.

Nutrition: Calories: 357 Fat: 15.2g Carbs: 5.2g Protein: 44.8g

Chicken Hearts

Preparation time: 15 minutes

Cooking time: 8 hours

Servings: 2 people

Ingredients:

- 2 pounds of chicken hearts

- 1 onion, sliced

- 1-pound mushrooms, sliced

- 4 garlic cloves, minced

- 1 tablespoon Dijon mustard

- 1 teaspoon salt, fresh ground pepper, each

- ½ tablespoon paprika

- ½ tablespoon cayenne pepper

- 1 cup chicken stock

- ¼ cup of coconut milk

- 7 oz. Greek yogurt, full fat

Directions:

1. Rinse the chicken, pat dry. Place all the ingredients, up to the chicken stock, in a slow cooker. Cover and cook on low within 8 hours.

2. Once finished cooking, stir in the cream and yogurt, wait 10 minutes and serve—side with potatoes, greens.

Nutrition:

Calories: 241

Fat: 11.8g

Carbs: 20.4g

Protein: 14.8g

Chicken Roux Gumbo

Preparation time: 10 minutes

Cooking time: 6 hours

Servings: 4 people

Ingredients:

- 1 lb. chicken thighs, cut into halves

- 1 tablespoon of vegetable oil

- 1 lb. smoky sausage, sliced, crispy, and crumbled.

- Salt and black pepper- to taste

Aromatics:

- 1 bell pepper, diced

- 2 quarts' chicken stock

- 15 oz. canned tomatoes, diced

- 1 celery stalk, diced

- salt to taste

- 4 garlic cloves, minced

- 1/2 lbs. okra, sliced

- 1 yellow onion, diced

- a dash tabasco sauce

For the roux:

- 1/2 cup of almond flour

- 1/4 cup of vegetable oil

- 1 teaspoon of Cajun spice

Directions:

1. Start by throwing all the ingredients except okra and roux ingredients into the slow cooker. Cover it and cook for 5 hours on low.

2. Stir in okra and cook for another 1 hour on low heat. Mix all the roux ingredients and add them to the slow cooker. Stir cook on high until the sauce thickens. Serve warm.

Nutrition: Calories: 604 Fat: 30.6g Carbs: 1.4g Protein: 54.6g

www.ingramcontent.com/pod-product-compliance
Lightning Source LLC
Chambersburg PA
CBHW071111030426

42336CB00013BA/2038